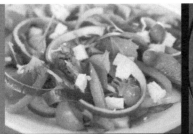
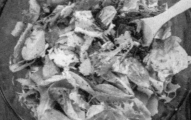
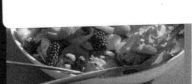

NEXT LEVEL
MENOPAUSE
COOKBOOK

275 Recipes Inspired by Stacy Sims to Boost Your Energy, Ease Symptoms, and Feel Your Best

Lily Mae Parker

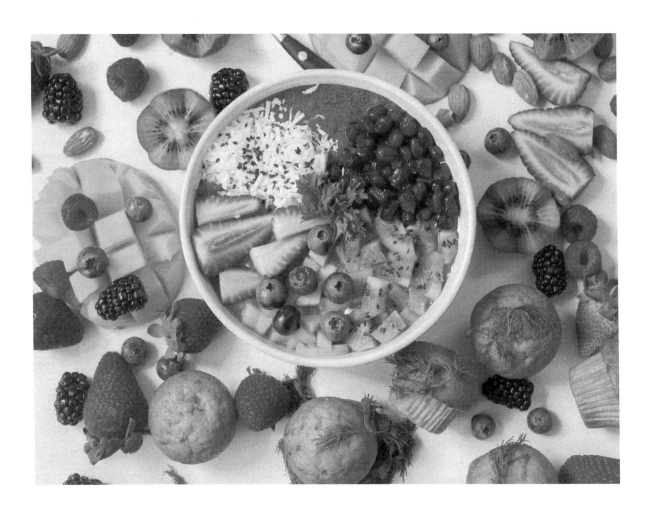

Table of Contents

Chapter 4: High-Protein, Low-Carb Lunches for Optimal Metabolism..48

Chapter 5: Hormone-Optimising Dinners Rich in Omega-3s and Antioxidants..62

Introduction

A few years ago, I met a woman named Karen. She was a force of nature—an avid cyclist, marathon runner, and yoga enthusiast. For most of her life, Karen had been used to pushing her limits, always aiming for her personal best. But then, something changed.

It wasn't overnight, but it felt that way to her. The workouts that used to feel exhilarating suddenly left her exhausted. The pounds seemed to creep up, no matter how clean she ate or how long she ran. Recovery times stretched longer, and she couldn't seem to bounce back after a hard training session like she used to. Hot flashes interrupted her sleep, zapping her energy for the day ahead. Karen was frustrated, and even worse, she was scared. Had her body betrayed her? Was this just how it was going to be from now on?

If Karen's story sounds familiar, you're not alone. Menopause can feel like an unexpected roadblock, throwing everything you once knew about your body into disarray. One moment you're at the top of your game, and the next, your strength, endurance, and metabolism seem to vanish into thin air. As an active, driven woman, it's easy to feel like your body is working against you. But here's the good news: it doesn't have to be that way.

Menopause is a transition, not an ending. And in this book, we're going to take a deep dive into how you can work with the changes in your body—using the right nutrition, fitness strategies, and recovery tools to not just survive menopause, but thrive through it. Next Level Menopause Cookbook is here to help you regain control, find your new groove, and continue kicking ass at the gym, on the trail, in the saddle, or wherever you pursue your passion.

In these pages, you'll find the answers you've been looking for. We'll break down the hormonal shifts behind menopause so you can understand why your body feels different and what's happening under the surface.

Then, we'll show you how to support your body with the right foods—meals that nourish your muscles, balance your hormones, and boost your metabolism. You'll get actionable, science-backed advice on what to eat, when to eat, and how to adjust your meals based on your activity levels. Whether you're looking for energy-packed breakfasts, post-workout recovery dinners, or satisfying snacks that won't derail your progress, we've got you covered.

More importantly, this isn't just another generic health book. It's a guide designed for active women—women like Karen, women like you—who aren't ready to slow down just because your hormones are shifting. You're going to learn how to fuel your body so it can keep up with the demands of your active lifestyle, while also addressing the unique challenges menopause brings. This book will empower you to take charge of your health and stay at the top of your game, well into the next phase of life.

So, if you've been feeling out of sync with your body and wondering how to get back to feeling strong, energised, and unstoppable—know that this is your solution. The Next Level is within reach, and I'm here to help you get there.

Let's do this.

Understanding Menopause: The Transition to the Next Level

For many active women, menopause can feel like a sudden and unexpected roadblock. You're used to being in control of your body—whether through pushing yourself in the gym, running marathons, or practising yoga—but then, seemingly overnight, your body starts behaving in ways that feel unfamiliar. The workouts you used to power through with ease leave you feeling fatigued for days. You gain weight despite sticking to the same healthy diet you've followed for years. Recovery takes longer, your joints ache, and sleep becomes elusive.

Welcome to menopause—a natural, yet profound transition in a woman's life. Menopause is not just about the end of your menstrual cycles; it signals a broader transformation in how your body functions. It's often referred to as "the change," and for good reason. Menopause alters your hormones, metabolism, and physical capacity. But, it's important to recognize that menopause is not the end of your vitality, strength, or athleticism. It's simply a new chapter—one that requires a different approach to health, fitness, and nutrition.

This transition doesn't have to be frustrating, and it certainly doesn't mean that you need to hang up your running shoes or cut back on your workouts. Instead, menopause offers an opportunity to learn more about your body, embrace these changes, and adapt your lifestyle to continue thriving—whether that's in the gym, on the trail, or during your favourite yoga session. By understanding how your body is changing and knowing what adjustments to make, you can navigate menopause and remain active, strong, and energised well into your post-menopausal years.

How This Cookbook Can Support Active Women Through Menopause

The Next Level Menopause Cookbook is more than just a collection of recipes; it's a comprehensive guide for active women to optimise their health, performance, and well-being during and after menopause. This book is designed with the needs of athletic, fitness-focused women in mind—women who are determined to continue thriving through menopause, not just survive it.

Throughout this cookbook, you'll find science-backed advice, real-world solutions, and practical strategies that address the specific challenges menopause brings to active women. Whether it's managing weight, preserving muscle mass, or finding ways to fuel your workouts, the recipes and guidance provided in these pages are designed to help you meet your goals and adapt to your body's evolving needs.

Tailored Nutrition for Hormonal Balance

One of the most significant impacts of menopause is the change in hormone levels—particularly estrogen and progesterone. These hormones play a crucial role in metabolism, fat distribution, muscle maintenance, and even energy levels. As they fluctuate and eventually decline during menopause, it's common to experience symptoms like weight gain, muscle loss, fatigue, and changes in appetite.

The recipes in this cookbook are carefully crafted to support hormonal balance and help you manage these symptoms through nutrition. You'll find meals rich in the nutrients your body needs to thrive during menopause, such as lean proteins to preserve muscle, healthy fats to support hormone production, and fibre-rich carbohydrates to stabilise blood sugar levels.

By nourishing your body with the right foods, you can counteract many of the negative effects of hormonal changes and maintain your energy, strength, and performance.

Supporting Metabolism and Weight Management

As many women notice, menopause can lead to changes in how your body stores fat—especially around the midsection. This is primarily due to a decrease in estrogen, which influences fat distribution and metabolism. Many active women find that they start gaining weight during menopause, even if their exercise and eating habits haven't changed.

This cookbook offers a solution. By focusing on high-protein, low-carb recipes, along with meals that prioritise nutrient-dense ingredients, you can support your metabolism and prevent unwanted weight gain. The recipes are designed to help you stay full and satisfied while providing the essential nutrients your body needs to fuel workouts, preserve muscle, and maintain a healthy metabolism.

Enhanced Recovery and Performance

Recovery becomes even more important during menopause. With hormonal changes affecting everything from muscle repair to joint health, it's essential to prioritise recovery through proper nutrition. In this cookbook, you'll find recipes that include anti-inflammatory ingredients, healthy fats like omega-3s, and foods rich in antioxidants—all of which support faster recovery, reduce muscle soreness, and keep your joints feeling strong.

Additionally, this cookbook includes tips on pre- and post-workout nutrition, so you can fuel your body appropriately before you exercise and help it recover afterward. Whether you're looking for quick, energising snacks or hearty, recovery-boosting dinners, you'll find meals tailored to meet the needs of active women navigating menopause.

The Science Behind Menopause: Hormonal Changes, Symptoms, and Their Effects

Understanding the hormonal shifts that occur during menopause is key to managing the symptoms and challenges that come with this transition. Menopause marks the end of a woman's reproductive years, which involves a significant decline in the production of hormones like oestrogen and progesterone. These hormones play critical roles in various bodily functions, including metabolism, muscle health, fat storage, and overall energy levels.

The Role of Oestrogen and Progesterone

Oestrogen is often thought of as the primary hormone affected during menopause, and its decline has far-reaching effects on the body. Oestrogen helps regulate the body's metabolism, maintains bone density, and even influences the production of collagen, which is vital for skin elasticity and joint health. When oestrogen levels drop, it becomes harder to maintain muscle mass, recover from workouts, and keep bones strong—all of which are crucial for active women.

Progesterone, another hormone that decreases during menopause, also plays a role in regulating mood, sleep, and water retention. With lower progesterone levels, many women experience symptoms like mood swings, poor sleep quality, and bloating, all of which can hinder physical performance and well-being.

Impact on Metabolism and Weight Gain

Weight gain, especially around the abdomen, is a frequent concern during menopause, often due to hormonal changes, a slowing metabolism, and lifestyle factors. This is due to a combination of hormonal changes, including the decline in oestrogen, as well as age-related metabolic slowdown. As oestrogen decreases, the body tends to store more fat, especially visceral fat (fat that accumulates around the organs).

In addition, the loss of muscle mass that often occurs with ageing can further slow metabolism. Muscle tissue is more metabolically active than fat tissue, so when muscle is lost, the body's ability to burn calories decreases. This is why strength training, combined with the right nutrition, is crucial during menopause to preserve lean muscle and keep your metabolism firing.

Bone Health and Muscle Preservation

Another major concern during menopause is the loss of bone density, which can increase the risk of osteoporosis. Oestrogen helps maintain bone health, and its decline can lead to the gradual weakening of bones. This makes it essential for women to get enough calcium, vitamin D, and other bone-strengthening nutrients through their diet.

Muscle preservation is equally important. With age and hormonal changes, women tend to lose muscle mass, making it harder to maintain strength and endurance. The high-protein recipes in this cookbook are designed to help you preserve muscle tissue and support your workouts, ensuring that you stay strong and active even as your body transitions through menopause.

Menopause Symptoms and Their Impact on Performance

In addition to weight gain and muscle loss, menopause brings a range of symptoms that can affect athletic performance. Hot flashes, night sweats, and sleep disturbances can leave you feeling fatigued and less motivated to exercise. Mood swings and irritability can make it harder to stick to a fitness routine, while joint pain and stiffness can hinder your mobility and make recovery more difficult.

This cookbook addresses these symptoms head-on, providing nutritional solutions to help manage everything from hot flashes to poor sleep. By incorporating foods that reduce inflammation, balance blood sugar, and promote restful sleep, you'll be better equipped to handle the physical and emotional challenges of menopause.

Conclusion

Menopause may bring new challenges, but it also presents an opportunity to take your health and performance to the next level. By understanding the hormonal changes and their effects on your body, you can adapt your nutrition and fitness strategies to continue thriving. This cookbook is your guide to navigating this transition with strength, energy, and confidence—so you can keep doing the things you love, whether you're in the gym, on the trail, or enjoying a morning yoga session.

Chapter 1: Embracing Your New Physiology

Menopause is a natural part of a woman's life—a transition that brings about profound hormonal, physical, and emotional changes. While it's often perceived as a time of decline, this stage can also be seen as an opportunity to reframe your health and well-being. In this chapter, we will dive deep into the physiological changes that occur during menopause and how they impact your body's performance. More importantly, we will discuss how you can embrace these changes with a positive mindset, optimise your health, and remain strong, fit, and resilient.

Hormonal Shifts and Their Impact on Performance

The hallmark of menopause is the significant shift in hormones, particularly oestrogen, progesterone, and testosterone. Understanding how these hormones influence your body's performance is crucial to navigating this transition with confidence and grace.

The Role of Oestrogen

Oestrogen, one of the most important female hormones, begins to decline in the years leading up to menopause, a phase called perimenopause. Oestrogen plays a vital role in regulating many of the body's functions, including reproduction, bone health, metabolism, and even cognitive function. As oestrogen levels decrease, the body experiences a range of physical changes that can impact how you feel and perform.

Bone Health: Oestrogen is vital for supporting bone density. Its decline can lead to a loss of bone mass, increasing the risk of osteoporosis and fractures. This can have a significant impact on athletic performance, especially in weight-bearing activities like running, jumping, and lifting weights.

Cardiovascular Health: Oestrogen helps to protect the heart and blood vessels by maintaining healthy cholesterol levels and promoting good circulation. As oestrogen decreases, women become more susceptible to cardiovascular issues, which can affect stamina and endurance.

Muscle Mass and Recovery: Oestrogen also plays a role in muscle health. As it declines, you may notice a reduction in muscle mass, strength, and recovery time after workouts. This can make it more challenging to maintain the same level of fitness you had in your pre-menopausal years.

The Role of Progesterone

Progesterone, another key hormone that declines during menopause, is responsible for regulating menstruation and preparing the body for pregnancy. However, its influence goes beyond reproduction.

Sleep and Mood Regulation: Progesterone has a calming effect on the body and supports restful sleep. As levels drop, many women experience sleep disturbances, insomnia, and increased anxiety, all of which can affect athletic performance and energy levels.

Water Retention and Bloating: Progesterone helps balance fluid levels in the body. With lower levels, women may experience more water retention, bloating, and discomfort, which can hinder physical activity and cause fluctuations in body weight.

The Role of Testosterone

Though often associated with men, testosterone plays an important role in women's health as well. It supports muscle growth, strength, and libido. As women age and testosterone levels decline, maintaining muscle mass and physical strength becomes more challenging.

Muscle and Strength: Testosterone contributes to the development of lean muscle mass. During menopause, as testosterone declines, it becomes more difficult to build and maintain muscle tissue. This can affect your overall strength and performance in activities like weightlifting, cycling, or running.

Energy Levels: Testosterone also influences energy levels and motivation. With lower levels, many women feel more fatigued and less driven to maintain an active lifestyle. This can make it harder to stay consistent with workouts or maintain previous levels of physical performance.

How Menopause Affects Metabolism, Muscle, and Fat Distribution

With the hormonal shifts that occur during menopause, the body's metabolism undergoes significant changes. These changes can be frustrating, particularly for active women who have spent years building strength and fitness. However, understanding how menopause affects metabolism, muscle mass, and fat distribution will help you better navigate this transition and adapt your nutrition and exercise routines.

Metabolic Slowdown

One of the most common complaints during menopause is the gradual slowdown of metabolism. This is largely due to the loss of oestrogen, which helps regulate how the body burns calories and stores fat. As oestrogen declines, the body becomes less efficient at burning calories, even at rest. This metabolic slowdown can lead to weight gain, even in women who continue to exercise and eat well.

Impact on Weight Maintenance: The body's ability to maintain a healthy weight becomes more challenging post-menopause. Even with the same level of activity and caloric intake, many women notice a gradual increase in body fat, particularly around the midsection.

Adjusting Caloric Intake: With a slower metabolism, it becomes essential to adjust your caloric intake and focus on nutrient-dense foods that support your energy needs without contributing to excess fat storage. Incorporating more protein, fibre, and healthy fats into your diet can help manage weight gain and keep your metabolism functioning optimally.

Muscle Loss (Sarcopenia)

Muscle loss, also known as sarcopenia, is another significant issue women face during menopause. As both oestrogen and testosterone levels decline, the body's ability to build and maintain muscle mass diminishes.

Preserving Lean Muscle: Muscle is metabolically active tissue, meaning it helps the body burn more calories at rest. The loss of muscle mass not only affects physical strength and performance but also contributes to the metabolic slowdown mentioned earlier. To counteract this, strength training becomes crucial during menopause. Incorporating resistance exercises like weightlifting, bodyweight exercises, and resistance bands can help preserve lean muscle mass and support a healthy metabolism.

Protein Intake: Nutrition plays a vital role in muscle preservation. Consuming adequate amounts of protein is essential for muscle repair and growth. Aim to include high-quality protein sources, such as lean meats, eggs, fish, tofu, and legumes, in each meal to support muscle maintenance and recovery.

Changes in Fat Distribution

One of the most noticeable changes during menopause is the shift in fat distribution. Many women who previously carried weight in their hips and thighs notice that fat begins to accumulate around the midsection, leading to the infamous "menopausal belly." This change is due to the decrease in oestrogen, which affects where the body stores fat.

Visceral Fat: Fat gained during menopause is often visceral fat, which accumulates around the abdominal organs and can increase the risk of cardiovascular disease, diabetes, and other health issues. Unlike subcutaneous fat (the fat stored under the skin), visceral fat is more metabolically active and can be harder to lose.

Managing Fat Distribution: To manage changes in fat distribution, it's important to focus on both diet and exercise. High-intensity interval training (HIIT) and strength training can be particularly effective in reducing visceral fat and improving overall body composition. Additionally, adopting a diet rich in whole, unprocessed foods, fibre, and healthy fats can help minimise fat gain and promote a leaner physique.

Building a Positive Mindset for Your Next Chapter

As your body changes during menopause, it's easy to feel discouraged, frustrated, or even defeated. However, it's important to remember that menopause is not an end—it's simply a transition into a new phase of life. By adopting a positive mindset, you can continue to thrive and embrace the opportunities that this stage brings.

Reframing Menopause as a New Beginning

Rather than viewing menopause as a loss or decline, it can be empowering to reframe it as a new beginning. Menopause marks the end of reproductive years, but it also brings newfound freedom and possibilities. Without the demands of monthly cycles, pregnancy, or birth control, you have the opportunity to focus more on your personal goals, health, and well-being.

Shifting Focus: Instead of dwelling on what your body can no longer do, focus on what it can still achieve. You may need to adjust your approach to fitness and nutrition, but that doesn't mean you can't continue to perform at a high level. Celebrate your body for its strength, resilience, and adaptability.

Setting New Goals: As you enter this new chapter, consider setting new health and fitness goals that align with your body's changing needs. These goals may focus on maintaining strength, improving flexibility, enhancing cardiovascular health, or simply feeling more energised and confident. Setting realistic, achievable goals will help you stay motivated and engaged with your fitness routine.

Embracing Self-Compassion

Menopause can bring about physical and emotional challenges, and it's important to practise self-compassion during this time. It's natural to feel frustrated with the changes your body is undergoing, but beating yourself up or comparing yourself to your younger self won't serve you. Instead, approach this transition with kindness and patience.

Listening to Your Body: Pay attention to your body's cues and recognize when it needs rest, nourishment, or a different approach to exercise. Pushing yourself too hard or ignoring signs of fatigue can lead to burnout and injury. By listening to your body and respecting its limits, you'll be better equipped to adapt to these changes in a healthy way.

Celebrating Small Wins: Progress during menopause may look different from what you're used to, but it's still worth celebrating. Whether it's completing a challenging workout, improving your sleep, or maintaining a consistent fitness routine, acknowledge your efforts and take pride in the small victories along the way.

Finding Support and Community

Navigating menopause can be easier when you have a supportive community around you. Whether it's through fitness groups, online forums, or close friends who are going through similar experiences, finding others who understand the challenges of menopause can provide valuable encouragement and motivation.

Sharing Experiences: Don't be afraid to talk openly about menopause and the changes you're experiencing. Sharing your journey with others can help normalise the conversation around menopause and empower other women to embrace their own transitions.

Seeking Professional Guidance: If you're struggling with certain aspects of menopause, such as weight gain, sleep disturbances, or emotional changes, consider seeking guidance from professionals such as a nutritionist, personal trainer, or therapist. Having expert support can make the transition smoother and ensure that you're taking the best possible care of your body and mind.

Conclusion

Menopause is a time of significant change, but it doesn't have to be a time of decline. By understanding the hormonal shifts and their impact on performance, adapting your approach to nutrition and exercise, and cultivating a positive mindset, you can navigate this transition with confidence and grace. Embrace your new physiology, celebrate your strength, and continue to thrive in this exciting new chapter of life.

Chapter 2: Fitness and Nutrition Through the Transition

As women go through menopause, their bodies undergo profound changes that impact every facet of their health—physical, mental, and emotional. While menopause is often accompanied by challenges such as weight gain, fatigue, and mood fluctuations, it also presents an opportunity to adjust your approach to fitness and nutrition in ways that support long-term health and well-being. In this chapter, we will explore why exercise needs to evolve post-menopause, the critical role nutrition plays in managing menopause symptoms, and the importance of sleep, recovery, and supplementation in this transformative phase.

Why Exercise Needs to Evolve Post-Menopause

During menopause, hormonal fluctuations—primarily the decline of oestrogen—have a direct impact on muscle mass, bone density, metabolism, and cardiovascular health. For active women, this can result in reduced strength, endurance, and recovery ability. However, rather than seeing menopause as a time to slow down, it's the perfect time to adapt and evolve your exercise routine to meet your body's changing needs.

Addressing Muscle Loss and Maintaining Strength

One of the most significant changes during menopause is the loss of muscle mass, also known as sarcopenia. This occurs due to the drop in oestrogen and testosterone, both of which are crucial for muscle repair and growth. Sarcopenia not only affects physical strength but also reduces your resting metabolic rate, making it easier to gain fat and harder to maintain a healthy weight.

Strength Training Becomes Essential: To counteract muscle loss, strength training is non-negotiable for post-menopausal women. Lifting weights, using resistance bands, or performing bodyweight exercises (like squats, lunges, and push-ups) helps preserve lean muscle mass, boosts metabolism, and enhances functional strength. Aim for at least two to three strength training sessions per week, focusing on all major muscle groups. Progressive overload—gradually increasing the weight or resistance used—ensures continued muscle growth and maintenance.

Incorporating Compound Movements: Exercises that engage multiple muscle groups at once, such as deadlifts, bench presses, and pull-ups, are particularly effective for building strength and stability. These compound movements mimic real-life activities and improve overall functionality, balance, and coordination, which are especially important as you age.

Supporting Bone Health

With the decline in estrogen, post-menopausal women are at a higher risk of osteoporosis, a condition in which bones become weak and brittle. Strength training not only builds muscle but also strengthens bones, helping to mitigate the loss of bone density that accompanies menopause.

Weight-Bearing Activities: Activities that place stress on the bones—such as walking, running, dancing, or hiking—are critical for maintaining bone health. These exercises force your bones to adapt by becoming stronger. High-impact activities like jumping or skipping may be beneficial for bone density, but always consider your joint health and individual fitness level when incorporating high-impact exercises.

Flexibility and Balance Training: Menopause can affect joint flexibility and balance due to hormonal changes. Incorporating flexibility exercises like yoga, Pilates, or simple stretching routines can improve joint mobility and reduce stiffness. Balance exercises, such as standing on one leg or using a balance board, help reduce the risk of falls, which can become more common as bone density decreases.

Cardiovascular Health and Metabolism

Menopause also increases the risk of cardiovascular disease, partly because oestrogen has a protective effect on the heart. Oestrogen helps maintain healthy blood vessels and cholesterol levels. As oestrogen levels drop, women become more vulnerable to high blood pressure, high cholesterol, and other cardiovascular issues. At the same time, the metabolic slowdown makes it more difficult to manage weight and maintain the same level of fitness.

Focus on Heart Health: Cardiovascular exercise remains a key component of a well-rounded fitness routine, but it may need to be tailored to reflect changes in endurance and metabolism. Activities like brisk walking, cycling, swimming, or interval training can boost heart health, burn calories, and help maintain a healthy weight. Aim for at least 150 minutes of moderate-intensity cardio or 75 minutes of vigorous-intensity cardio per week to keep your heart strong and support metabolism.

High-Intensity Interval Training (HIIT): For women experiencing a slower metabolism, high-intensity interval training (HIIT) can be a game-changer. HIIT consists of brief, high-intensity exercises alternated with intervals of rest or reduced intensity.

This type of training not only improves cardiovascular health but also increases calorie burn during and after workouts, thanks to the "afterburn effect" (excess post-exercise oxygen consumption). HIIT sessions can be tailored to individual fitness levels, making them suitable for women of all ages and abilities.

Prioritising Recovery

Menopause can slow down the body's ability to recover from workouts due to hormonal changes that affect muscle repair and inflammation. To prevent injury and burnout, recovery needs to be an integral part of your fitness regimen.

Active Recovery: Incorporating active recovery days, where you engage in light activities like walking, swimming, or yoga, helps maintain circulation, reduce stiffness, and promote muscle repair without overexerting yourself.

Rest Days: Adequate rest is just as important as exercise itself. Post-menopausal women need to be mindful of not overtraining, which can lead to chronic fatigue, injury, and elevated cortisol levels (the stress hormone). Listen to your body's cues and allow for full rest days when needed.

The Impact of Diet on Alleviating Menopause Symptoms

As menopause brings metabolic changes, muscle loss, and weight gain, nutrition plays a critical role in managing symptoms and optimising overall health. With the right dietary choices, women can balance hormones, maintain muscle, support bone health, and reduce the risk of chronic diseases that are more common after menopause.

Protein for Muscle Maintenance

Protein becomes increasingly important during menopause due to the loss of muscle mass. Without enough protein, the body struggles to repair and build muscle, which can exacerbate muscle loss.

Increase Protein Intake: To support muscle maintenance, aim to consume 1.0 to 1.2 grams of protein per kilogram of body weight per day. High-quality protein sources include lean meats, fish, poultry, eggs, dairy, tofu, and legumes. Protein is also crucial for recovery after exercise, so make sure to include protein-rich meals and snacks throughout the day.

Distribute Protein Evenly: Instead of consuming most of your protein at dinner, try to distribute it evenly across all meals. This approach maximises muscle protein synthesis and helps maintain lean muscle mass over time.

Healthy Fats for Hormonal Balance

During menopause, incorporating healthy fats into your diet can help balance hormones and reduce inflammation, which is particularly important for managing symptoms like hot flashes, mood swings, and joint pain.

Omega-3 Fatty Acids: Omega-3 fatty acids, found in fatty fish (such as salmon, mackerel, and sardines), flaxseeds, chia seeds, and walnuts, play a key role in reducing inflammation and supporting heart health. These fats may also help alleviate some of the mood-related symptoms of menopause, such as anxiety and depression.

Monounsaturated Fats: Avocados, olive oil, and nuts are rich in monounsaturated fats, which can support cardiovascular health and help regulate hormone production.

Avoid Trans Fats: It's important to avoid trans fats and processed foods, which can increase inflammation and contribute to weight gain, particularly around the abdomen, where fat tends to accumulate during menopause.

Fibre for Digestive Health and Weight Management

Menopause can slow down digestion and lead to bloating and constipation. A diet rich in fibre helps promote digestive health, stabilise blood sugar levels, and support weight management.

Increase Fibre Intake: Include high-fibre foods such as vegetables, fruits, whole grains, legumes, and seeds in your diet. These foods not only promote gut health but also help you feel fuller for longer, reducing the likelihood of overeating.

Soluble and Insoluble Fibre: Both types of fibre are beneficial. Soluble fibre (found in oats, apples, and beans) helps manage cholesterol and blood sugar levels, while insoluble fibre (found in whole grains and vegetables) promotes regular bowel movements.

Calcium and Vitamin D for Bone Health

The loss of oestrogen during menopause accelerates the breakdown of bone tissue, increasing the risk of osteoporosis. Adequate calcium and vitamin D intake are essential for maintaining strong bones and preventing fractures.

Calcium-Rich Foods: Aim for 1,200 mg of calcium per day through foods such as dairy products (milk, yoghourt, and cheese), leafy green vegetables, fortified plant-based milks, and tofu. If you struggle to meet your calcium needs through food alone, a supplement may be necessary.

Vitamin D for Absorption: Vitamin D helps the body absorb calcium effectively. You can obtain vitamin D from sunlight, fortified foods, and supplements. If you live in a region with limited sunlight, consider getting your vitamin D levels checked to determine if supplementation is needed.

Phytoestrogens for Hormonal Support

Phytoestrogens are naturally occurring plant compounds that act similarly to oestrogen in the body. Research indicates that they may provide relief from menopausal symptoms such as hot flashes and night sweats.

Sources of Phytoestrogens: Soy products (such as tofu, tempeh, and edamame), flaxseeds, sesame seeds, and lentils are rich in phytoestrogens. Including these foods in your diet may provide mild relief from hormone-related symptoms, though their effectiveness varies from person to person.

Importance of Sleep, Recovery, and Supplementation

Menopause often disrupts sleep, which in turn affects energy levels, mood, and recovery from exercise. Prioritising rest, recovery, and supplementation can make a significant difference in your overall well-being.

Sleep and Hormone Regulation

Sleep disturbances are common during menopause, largely due to hot flashes and night sweats caused by hormonal fluctuations. Poor sleep can lead to increased cortisol levels, reduced insulin sensitivity, and difficulty maintaining a healthy weight.

Create a Sleep-Friendly Environment: Keep your bedroom cool, dark, and quiet. Create a calming bedtime routine by engaging in activities like reading, practising meditation, or enjoying a warm bath to promote relaxation before sleep. Avoid caffeine, alcohol, and heavy meals before bedtime, as they can disrupt sleep.

Consider Cognitive Behavioral Therapy (CBT): CBT for insomnia has been shown to be effective in improving sleep quality in menopausal women. CBT addresses the thoughts and behaviours that interfere with sleep, helping you develop healthier sleep patterns over time.

Recovery and Stress Management

Recovery is critical for maintaining overall health and fitness during menopause. Inadequate recovery can lead to overtraining, chronic fatigue, and increased stress levels, which negatively impact hormone balance.

Incorporate Relaxation Techniques: Stress reduction is essential for managing cortisol levels, which can exacerbate menopause symptoms. Consider practices such as deep breathing exercises, yoga, or meditation to manage stress and promote relaxation.

Stay Hydrated: Proper hydration supports digestion, muscle recovery, and temperature regulation. Drink plenty of water throughout the day, especially before and after exercise, to stay hydrated and prevent dehydration-related fatigue.

Supplementation for Optimal Health

In addition to a nutrient-dense diet, supplementation can help address specific deficiencies or support areas of health that are particularly vulnerable during menopause.

Multivitamin: A high-quality multivitamin designed for women can help fill nutritional gaps, particularly if you struggle to get all the essential vitamins and minerals from your diet alone.

Magnesium: Magnesium supports muscle relaxation, reduces cramping, and promotes restful sleep. Many women benefit from magnesium supplementation to ease menopause-related symptoms, such as insomnia and anxiety.

Adaptogens: Herbal supplements like ashwagandha, maca root, and Rhodiola rosea are known for their ability to balance hormones, reduce stress, and enhance energy levels. While more research is needed, some women find adaptogens helpful in managing menopause symptoms.

As you transition through menopause, staying active and prioritising proper nutrition, sleep, and recovery are key to maintaining your health, strength, and vitality. By adjusting your fitness routine to support muscle and bone health, optimising your diet for hormonal balance, and ensuring you get adequate rest, you can navigate this life stage with confidence and grace. Remember, menopause is not the end—it's a powerful new beginning.

Chapter 3: Breakfasts for Energy and Hormone Balance

Avocado and Egg Toast

Ingredients (Serves 1):

1 slice whole-grain bread

½ avocado

1 large egg

1 tsp olive oil

Salt and pepper to taste

1 tbsp chia seeds

Preparation Method:

Toast the slice of whole-grain bread until golden brown.

While the bread is toasting, heat the olive oil in a non-stick skillet over medium heat.

Crack the egg into the skillet and cook to your desired doneness (sunny-side-up, over-easy, etc.).

Get the avocado mashed in a bowl and season with salt and pepper.

Get the mashed avocado spread on the toasted bread.

Get the cooked egg placed on top of the avocado toast.

Sprinkle chia seeds over the egg and serve immediately.

Nutritional Information:

Calories: 350 kcal

Protein: 13 g

Fat: 24 g

Carbohydrates: 23 g

Fibre: 8 g

Hormone-Balancing Smoothie

Ingredients (Serves 1):

1 cup unsweetened almond milk

½ banana

1 tbsp flaxseeds

1 tbsp almond butter

½ cup spinach

1 scoop protein powder (plant-based or whey)

1 tsp maca powder

Preparation Method:

Add all ingredients to a blender.

Have them blended on high speed until smooth and creamy.

Pour the smoothie into a glass and enjoy.

Nutritional Information:

Calories: 350 kcal

Protein: 22 g

Fat: 15 g

Carbohydrates: 34 g

Fibre: 8 g

Chia Pudding with Berries

Ingredients (Serves 2):

¼ cup chia seeds

1 cup unsweetened almond milk

1 tsp vanilla extract

1 tbsp maple syrup (optional)

½ cup mixed berries (blueberries, raspberries)

Preparation Method:

In a bowl, combine chia seeds, almond milk, vanilla extract, and maple syrup (if using).

Stir well to combine and let sit for 5 minutes. Stir again to prevent clumping.

Cover and have it refrigerated for at least 2 hours or overnight.

Serve topped with mixed berries.

Nutritional Information (per serving):

Calories: 220 kcal

Protein: 6 g

Fat: 12 g

Carbohydrates: 28 g

Fibre: 11 g

Sweet Potato and Spinach Frittata

Ingredients (Serves 4):

1 medium sweet potato, peeled and diced

2 cups spinach, chopped

6 large eggs

¼ cup feta cheese

1 tbsp olive oil

Salt and pepper to taste

Preparation Method:

Preheat the oven to 375°F (190°C).

In a skillet, heat olive oil over medium heat and add diced sweet potato. Cook for about 10 minutes until tender.

Add chopped spinach and cook until wilted.

In a bowl, whisk together eggs, salt, pepper, and crumbled feta.

Have the egg mixture poured over the vegetables in the skillet and stir gently.

Get the skillet transfered to the preheated oven and bake for 15-20 minutes or until the eggs are set.

Nutritional Information (per serving):

Calories: 220 kcal

Protein: 12 g

Fat: 13 g

Carbohydrates: 15 g

Fibre: 3 g

Oatmeal with Flaxseeds and Almonds

Ingredients (Serves 1):

½ cup rolled oats

1 cup water or almond milk

1 tbsp ground flaxseeds

10 almonds, chopped

1 tsp cinnamon

1 tsp honey (optional)

Preparation Method:

In a saucepan, have a water or almond milk boiled.

Add rolled oats and reduce the heat. Simmer for about 5 minutes until thickened.

Stir in ground flaxseeds and cinnamon.

Transfer oatmeal to a bowl and top with chopped almonds and honey, if desired.

Nutritional Information:

Calories: 300 kcal

Protein: 9 g

Fat: 13 g

Carbohydrates: 37 g

Fibre: 8 g

Greek Yogurt Parfait with Granola

Ingredients (Serves 1):

1 cup plain Greek yoghourt

¼ cup granola (low sugar)

½ cup mixed berries

1 tbsp chia seeds

1 tsp honey (optional)

Preparation Method:

In a bowl or a jar, layer the Greek yoghourt, granola, and mixed berries.

Sprinkle chia seeds on top of the layers.

Drizzle with honey if desired.

Nutritional Information:

Calories: 320 kcal

Protein: 20 g

Fat: 8 g

Carbohydrates: 44 g

Fibre: 9 g

Quinoa Breakfast Bowl with Eggs

Ingredients (Serves 2):

1 cup cooked quinoa

2 large eggs

½ avocado, sliced

1 tbsp olive oil

1 tbsp nutritional yeast

Salt and pepper to taste

Preparation Method:

Divide cooked quinoa into two bowls.

In a skillet, heat olive oil and fry the eggs until cooked to your preference.

Place the eggs on top of the quinoa in each bowl.

Top with sliced avocado and nutritional yeast.

Season with salt and pepper before serving.

Nutritional Information (per serving):

Calories: 350 kcal

Protein: 14 g

Fat: 22 g

Carbohydrates: 29 g

Fibre: 6 g

Whole Wheat Pancakes with Ground Flaxseeds

Ingredients (Serves 2):

½ cup whole wheat flour

1 tbsp ground flaxseeds

1 tsp baking powder

½ cup unsweetened almond milk

1 egg

1 tsp vanilla extract

1 tbsp coconut oil (for cooking)

Preparation Method:

In a bowl, get the whole wheat flour, ground flaxseeds, and baking powder combined.

In another bowl, mix almond milk, egg, and vanilla extract.

Have the wet and dry ingredients combined and stir until smooth.

Have coconut oil heated in a skillet over medium heat.

Pour batter onto the skillet to form pancakes and cook until bubbles form, then flip and cook until golden brown.

Nutritional Information (per serving):

Calories: 250 kcal

Protein: 9 g

Fat: 11 g

Carbohydrates: 30 g

Fibre: 6 g

Tofu Scramble with Vegetables

Ingredients (Serves 2):

200g firm tofu, crumbled

1 tbsp olive oil

½ cup bell peppers, chopped

½ cup mushrooms, sliced

¼ tsp turmeric

Salt and pepper to taste

1 tbsp nutritional yeast

Preparation Method:

Have the olive oil heated in a pan over medium heat.

Add chopped bell peppers and mushrooms, cooking until soft.

Stir in crumbled tofu and season with turmeric, salt, and pepper.

Cook for 5-7 minutes, stirring occasionally.

Sprinkle nutritional yeast on top and serve hot.

Nutritional Information (per serving):

Calories: 220 kcal

Protein: 15 g

Fat: 14 g

Carbohydrates: 12 g

Fibre: 4 g

Spinach and Mushroom Omelette

Ingredients (Serves 1):

2 large eggs

1 cup spinach, chopped

½ cup mushrooms, sliced

1 tbsp olive oil

Salt and pepper to taste

Preparation Method:

Heat olive oil in a skillet over medium heat.

Add sliced mushrooms and cook until softened.

Add spinach and cook until wilted.

In a bowl, whisk eggs with salt and pepper.

Pour the eggs over the vegetables and cook until set, gently folding the omelette in half.

Nutritional Information:

Calories: 250 kcal

Protein: 14 g

Fat: 19 g

Carbohydrates: 5 g

Fibre: 2 g

Overnight Oats with Almond Butter

Ingredients (Serves 1):

½ cup rolled oats

1 cup unsweetened almond milk

1 tbsp almond butter

1 tbsp chia seeds

1 tsp honey (optional)

½ banana, sliced

Preparation Method:

In a jar or bowl, combine rolled oats, almond milk, almond butter, chia seeds, and honey (if using).

Stir well, cover, and refrigerate overnight.

In the morning, have the oat topped with sliced banana before serving.

Nutritional Information:

Calories: 400 kcal

Protein: 13 g

Fat: 20 g

Carbohydrates: 46 g

Fibre: 10 g

Banana Oatmeal Muffins

Ingredients (Makes 12 muffins):

2 ripe bananas, mashed

1 cup rolled oats

½ cup almond milk

1 tsp baking powder

1 tsp cinnamon

¼ cup honey or maple syrup

1 tsp vanilla extract

Preparation Method:

Preheat the oven to 350°F (175°C) and have a muffin tin lined with liners.

In a bowl, combine mashed bananas, rolled oats, almond milk, baking powder, cinnamon, honey (or maple syrup), and vanilla extract.

Mix until well combined and spoon the batter into muffin tins.

Bake for about twenty five minutes or until a toothpick comes out clean.

Nutritional Information (per muffin):

Calories: 120 kcal

Protein: 3 g

Fat: 1 g

Carbohydrates: 26 g

Fibre: 3 g

Savory Quinoa Breakfast Bowl

Ingredients (Serves 1):

½ cup cooked quinoa

1 large egg

1 cup kale, chopped

1 tbsp olive oil

Salt and pepper to taste

1 tbsp pumpkin seeds

Preparation Method:

In a skillet, have olive oil heated over medium heat.

Add chopped kale and sauté until wilted.

In a separate pan, cook the egg to your preference (fried or poached).

In a bowl, layer the cooked quinoa, sautéed kale, and the cooked egg.

Sprinkle with pumpkin seeds, salt, and pepper before serving.

Nutritional Information:

Calories: 300 kcal

Protein: 13 g

Fat: 18 g

Carbohydrates: 26 g

Fibre: 5 g

Peanut Butter Banana Toast

Ingredients (Serves 1):

1 slice whole-grain bread

2 tbsp natural peanut butter

½ banana, sliced

1 tsp chia seeds

Preparation Method:

Get the slice of whole-grain bread toasted until golden brown.

Spread peanut butter evenly over the toast.

Top with banana slices and sprinkle chia seeds on top.

Nutritional Information:

Calories: 290 kcal

Protein: 11 g

Fat: 16 g

Carbohydrates: 29 g

Fibre: 5 g

Apple Cinnamon Quinoa

Ingredients (Serves 1):

½ cup cooked quinoa

½ apple, diced

1 tsp cinnamon

1 tbsp maple syrup

1 tbsp walnuts, chopped

Preparation Method:

In a bowl, combine cooked quinoa, diced apple, cinnamon, and maple syrup.

Stir to combine and warm in the microwave if desired.

Top with chopped walnuts before serving.

Nutritional Information:

Calories: 280 kcal

Protein: 6 g

Fat: 8 g

Carbohydrates: 48 g

Fiber: 5 g

Chapter 4: High-Protein, Low-Carb Lunches for Optimal Metabolism

Grilled Chicken Salad

Ingredients (Serves 2):

2 grilled chicken breasts (6 oz each)

4 cups mixed greens (spinach, arugula, romaine)

1 cup cherry tomatoes, halved

½ cucumber, sliced

¼ cup feta cheese, crumbled

2 tbsp olive oil

1 tbsp balsamic vinegar

Salt and pepper to taste

Preparation Method:

Slice the grilled chicken breasts and set aside.

In a large bowl, combine mixed greens, cherry tomatoes, cucumber, and feta cheese.

In a small bowl, get the olive oil, balsamic vinegar, salt, and pepper whisked together.

Toss the salad with the dressing and top with sliced chicken.

Nutritional Information (per serving):

Calories: 350 kcal

Protein: 40 g

Fat: 22 g

Carbohydrates: 8 g

Fibre: 3 g

Turkey and Avocado Lettuce Wraps

Ingredients (Serves 2):

8 slices turkey breast (deli meat)

1 avocado, sliced

4 large lettuce leaves (romaine or iceberg)

½ red bell pepper, sliced

2 tbsp mustard

Preparation Method:

Get the lettuce leaves laid out on a flat surface.

Spread mustard on each lettuce leaf.

Layer turkey slices, avocado, and red bell pepper.

Roll the lettuce leaves tightly and secure with toothpicks if necessary.

Nutritional Information (per serving):

Calories: 290 kcal

Protein: 28 g

Fat: 18 g

Carbohydrates: 8 g

Fibre: 5 g

Egg Salad with Greek Yoghourt

Ingredients (Serves 2):

4 hard-boiled eggs, chopped

¼ cup plain Greek yoghourt

1 tbsp Dijon mustard

1 tbsp fresh dill, chopped

Salt and pepper to taste

4 large romaine leaves for serving

Preparation Method:

In a bowl, combine chopped eggs, Greek yoghourt, Dijon mustard, dill, salt, and pepper.

Mix well until all ingredients are incorporated.

Serve on romaine leaves as wraps or with a fork.

Nutritional Information (per serving):

Calories: 250 kcal

Protein: 18 g

Fat: 15 g

Carbohydrates: 3 g

Fibre: 0 g

Shrimp Stir-Fry

Ingredients (Serves 2):

1 lb shrimp, peeled and deveined

2 cups broccoli florets

1 cup bell peppers, sliced

2 tbsp soy sauce

1 tbsp olive oil

1 tsp garlic powder

Salt and pepper to taste

Preparation Method:

In a skillet, have the olive oil heated over medium heat.

Have the shrimp added and cook until pink, about 3-4 minutes.

Add broccoli, bell peppers, soy sauce, garlic powder, salt, and pepper.

Stir-fry for an additional 5 minutes until vegetables are tender.

Nutritional Information (per serving):

Calories: 300 kcal

Protein: 40 g

Fat: 12 g

Carbohydrates: 8 g

Fibre: 3 g

Zucchini Noodles with Pesto Chicken

Ingredients (Serves 2):

2 medium zucchinis, spiralized

2 grilled chicken breasts (6 oz each), sliced

½ cup basil pesto

1 tbsp olive oil

Salt and pepper to taste

Parmesan cheese for topping (optional)

Preparation Method:

In a skillet, have the olive oil heated over medium heat.

Add zucchini noodles and sauté for 2-3 minutes until tender.

Stir in pesto and cooked chicken until heated through.

Serve with Parmesan cheese, if desired.

Nutritional Information (per serving):

Calories: 360 kcal

Protein: 40 g

Fat: 24 g

Carbohydrates: 8 g

Fibre: 3 g

Tuna Salad Stuffed Peppers

Ingredients (Serves 2):

1 can (5 oz) tuna in water, drained

¼ cup plain Greek yogurt

1 tbsp Dijon mustard

2 large bell peppers, halved and seeded

1 tbsp capers (optional)

Salt and pepper to taste

Preparation Method:

In a bowl, mix together tuna, Greek yoghourt, Dijon mustard, capers, salt, and pepper.

Have the tuna mixture spooned into the halved bell peppers.

Serve chilled or at room temperature.

Nutritional Information (per serving):

Calories: 240 kcal

Protein: 28 g

Fat: 7 g

Carbohydrates: 10 g

Fibre: 3 g

Beef and Broccoli

Ingredients (Serves 2):

8 oz flank steak, sliced thin

2 cups broccoli florets

2 tbsp soy sauce

1 tbsp sesame oil

1 tsp garlic, minced

1 tsp ginger, minced

1 tsp cornstarch (optional)

Preparation Method:

In a skillet, heat sesame oil over medium-high heat.

Add garlic, ginger, and sliced beef; cook until beef is browned.

Add broccoli and soy sauce; stir-fry for another 5 minutes until broccoli is tender.

If desired, mix cornstarch with a little water and add to thicken the sauce.

Nutritional Information (per serving):

Calories: 370 kcal

Protein: 42 g

Fat: 20 g

Carbohydrates: 10 g

Fibre: 3 g

Chicken Caesar Salad

Ingredients (Serves 2):

2 grilled chicken breasts (6 oz each), sliced

4 cups romaine lettuce, chopped

¼ cup Parmesan cheese, grated

¼ cup Caesar dressing (low-carb)

Black pepper to taste

Preparation Method:

In a large bowl, combine romaine lettuce and Caesar dressing.

Toss to coat evenly.

Top with sliced chicken and Parmesan cheese; season with black pepper.

Nutritional Information (per serving):

Calories: 380 kcal

Protein: 43 g

Fat: 23 g

Carbohydrates: 8 g

Fibre: 3 g

Eggplant Pizza Bites

Ingredients (Serves 2):

1 large eggplant, sliced into ½-inch rounds

1 cup marinara sauce (low-carb)

1 cup mozzarella cheese, shredded

1 tsp Italian seasoning

Salt and pepper to taste

Preparation Method:

Preheat the oven to 400°F (200°C).

Arrange eggplant slices on a baking sheet; season with salt and pepper.

Spread marinara sauce over each slice and top with mozzarella cheese.

Sprinkle with Italian seasoning and bake for 15-20 minutes until cheese is melted and bubbly.

Nutritional Information (per serving):

Calories: 220 kcal

Protein: 16 g

Fat: 14 g

Carbohydrates: 12 g

Fibre: 5 g

Salmon Avocado Salad

Ingredients (Serves 2):

2 salmon fillets (4 oz each)

1 avocado, diced

4 cups mixed greens

1 tbsp olive oil

1 tbsp lemon juice

Salt and pepper to taste

Preparation Method:

Grill or pan-sear the salmon fillets until cooked through.

In a bowl, combine mixed greens, diced avocado, olive oil, lemon juice, salt, and pepper.

Flake the salmon and add it to the salad; toss gently before serving.

Nutritional Information (per serving):

Calories: 410 kcal

Protein: 34 g

Fat: 28 g

Carbohydrates: 10 g

Fibre: 5 g

Cottage Cheese and Berry Bowl

Ingredients (Serves 2):

2 cups cottage cheese (low-fat)

1 cup mixed berries (strawberries, blueberries, raspberries)

2 tbsp chia seeds

1 tsp honey (optional)

Preparation Method:

In a bowl, divide cottage cheese between two serving bowls.

Top each with mixed berries and chia seeds.

Drizzle with honey if desired.

Nutritional Information (per serving):

Calories: 250 kcal

Protein: 28 g

Fat: 5 g

Carbohydrates: 22 g

Fibre: 7 g

Stuffed Portobello Mushrooms

Ingredients (Serves 2):

4 large Portobello mushrooms

1 cup cooked ground turkey (or beef)

1 cup spinach, chopped

½ cup marinara sauce (low-carb)

1 cup mozzarella cheese, shredded

1 tsp Italian seasoning

Preparation Method:

Preheat the oven to 375°F (190°C).

Clean Portobello mushrooms and remove stems.

In a bowl, mix cooked ground turkey, spinach, marinara sauce, and Italian seasoning.

Stuff the mushroom caps with the mixture and top with mozzarella cheese.

Bake for 25 minutes until mushrooms are tender.

Nutritional Information (per serving):

Calories: 320 kcal

Protein: 40 g

Fat: 15 g

Carbohydrates: 10 g

Fibre: 4 g

Chickpea Salad with Tuna

Ingredients (Serves 2):

One can (15 oz) of drained rinsed chickpeas

1 can (5 oz) tuna in water, drained

1 cup cherry tomatoes, halved

½ cucumber, diced

2 tbsp olive oil

1 tbsp lemon juice

Salt and pepper to taste

Preparation Method:

In a large bowl, combine chickpeas, tuna, cherry tomatoes, and cucumber.

Have olive oil and lemon juice drizzled, then season with salt and pepper.

Toss to combine and serve chilled.

Nutritional Information (per serving):

Calories: 350 kcal

Protein: 28 g

Fat: 14 g

Carbohydrates: 35 g

Fibre: 10 g

Sausage and Egg Muffins

Ingredients (Serves 2):

4 large eggs

1 cup cooked sausage (crumbled)

1 cup spinach, chopped

½ cup bell peppers, diced

Salt and pepper to taste

Preparation Method:

Preheat the oven to 350°F (175°C) and grease a muffin tin.

In a bowl, get the eggs whisked and season with salt and pepper.

Add sausage, spinach, and bell peppers to the egg mixture.

Pour the mixture into muffin cups, filling them halfway.

Bake for about twenty five minutes until muffins are set.

Nutritional Information (per serving):

Calories: 280 kcal

Protein: 22 g

Fat: 20 g

Carbohydrates: 4 g

Fiber: 1 g

Chapter 5: Hormone-Optimising Dinners Rich in Omega-3s and Antioxidants

Grilled Salmon with Avocado Salsa

Ingredients (Serves 2):

2 (6 oz) salmon fillets

1 avocado, diced

1 cup cherry tomatoes, halved

¼ red onion, finely chopped

2 tbsp lime juice

Salt and pepper to taste

Preparation Method:

Preheat the grill to medium-high heat.

Season salmon fillets with salt and pepper.

Grill salmon for about 5-6 minutes on each side until cooked through.

In a bowl, mix avocado, cherry tomatoes, red onion, lime juice, salt, and pepper.

Serve the grilled salmon topped with avocado salsa.

Nutritional Information (per serving):

Calories: 450 kcal

Protein: 40 g

Fat: 30 g

Carbohydrates: 10 g

Fibre: 7 g

Quinoa and Spinach Salad with Walnuts

Ingredients (Serves 2):

1 cup cooked quinoa

2 cups fresh spinach, chopped

¼ cup walnuts, chopped

¼ cup feta cheese, crumbled

2 tbsp olive oil

1 tbsp balsamic vinegar

Salt and pepper to taste

Preparation Method:

In a large bowl, combine cooked quinoa, spinach, walnuts, and feta cheese.

In a small bowl, get the olive oil, balsamic vinegar, salt, and pepper whisked together.

Have the dressing drizzled over the salad and toss to combine.

Nutritional Information (per serving):

Calories: 350 kcal

Protein: 12 g

Fat: 22 g

Carbohydrates: 32 g

Fibre: 5 g

Lentil and Sweet Potato Stew

Ingredients (Serves 4):

1 cup lentils, rinsed

1 large sweet potato, diced

1 can (14 oz) diced tomatoes

4 cups vegetable broth

1 onion, chopped

2 cloves garlic, minced

1 tsp cumin

1 tsp smoked paprika

Salt and pepper to taste

Preparation Method:

In a large pot, sauté onion and garlic until translucent.

Add sweet potato, lentils, diced tomatoes, vegetable broth, cumin, smoked paprika, salt, and pepper.

Bring to a boil, then have the heat minimised and simmer for 30-35 minutes until lentils and sweet potatoes are tender.

Nutritional Information (per serving):

Calories: 280 kcal

Protein: 15 g

Fat: 1 g

Carbohydrates: 55 g

Fibre: 15 g

Baked Mackerel with Lemon and Dill

Ingredients (Serves 2):

2 (6 oz) mackerel fillets

2 tbsp olive oil

1 lemon, sliced

2 tbsp fresh dill, chopped

Salt and pepper to taste

Preparation Method:

Preheat the oven to 400°F (200°C).

Place mackerel fillets on a baking sheet and drizzle with olive oil.

Top with lemon slices, dill, salt, and pepper.

Bake for about eighteen minutes until the fish flakes easily with a fork.

Nutritional Information (per serving):

Calories: 390 kcal

Protein: 36 g

Fat: 27 g

Carbohydrates: 2 g

Fibre: 0 g

Chickpea and Spinach Curry

Ingredients (Serves 4):

One can (15 oz) of drained and rinsed chickpeas

2 cups spinach, chopped

1 can (14 oz) coconut milk

1 onion, chopped

2 cloves garlic, minced

1 tbsp curry powder

Salt and pepper to taste

Preparation Method:

In a large pan, sauté onion and garlic until soft.

Add chickpeas, coconut milk, curry powder, salt, and pepper.

Simmer for 10 minutes, then stir in spinach and cook until wilted.

Nutritional Information (per serving):

Calories: 300 kcal

Protein: 12 g

Fat: 15 g

Carbohydrates: 36 g

Fibre: 10 g

Zucchini Noodles with Pesto and Grilled Shrimp

Ingredients (Serves 2):

2 medium zucchinis, spiralized

1 cup shrimp, peeled and deveined

¼ cup basil pesto

2 tbsp olive oil

Salt and pepper to taste

Preparation Method:

In a skillet, have the olive oil heated over medium heat. Add shrimp, seasoning with salt and pepper, and cook until pink (about 3-4 minutes).

Add spiralized zucchini and sauté for another 2-3 minutes.

Stir in pesto and serve immediately.

Nutritional Information (per serving):

Calories: 300 kcal

Protein: 25 g

Fat: 20 g

Carbohydrates: 8 g

Fibre: 3 g

Stuffed Bell Peppers with Quinoa and Turkey

Ingredients (Serves 2):

2 large bell peppers, halved and seeded

1 cup cooked quinoa

1 cup cooked ground turkey

1 can (14 oz) diced tomatoes

1 tsp Italian seasoning

½ cup mozzarella cheese, shredded

Preparation Method:

Preheat the oven to 375°F (190°C).

In a bowl, mix quinoa, ground turkey, diced tomatoes, Italian seasoning, salt, and pepper.

Stuff each bell pepper half with the mixture and place in a baking dish.

Top with mozzarella cheese and bake for about twenty five minutes.

Nutritional Information (per serving):

Calories: 360 kcal

Protein: 30 g

Fat: 15 g

Carbohydrates: 30 g

Fibre: 7 g

Cauliflower Fried Rice with Edamame

Ingredients (Serves 2):

4 cups cauliflower rice

1 cup edamame (shelled)

2 carrots, diced

2 green onions, sliced

2 cloves garlic, minced

2 tbsp soy sauce (low-sodium)

Preparation Method:

In a large skillet, sauté garlic and carrots until tender.

Add cauliflower rice and edamame, cooking for about 5-7 minutes.

Stir in soy sauce and green onions; cook for an additional 2 minutes.

Nutritional Information (per serving):

Calories: 220 kcal

Protein: 15 g

Fat: 8 g

Carbohydrates: 25 g

Fibre: 8 g

Turkey and Spinach Stuffed Portobello Mushrooms

Ingredients (Serves 2):

4 large Portobello mushrooms

1 cup cooked ground turkey

2 cups spinach, chopped

½ cup ricotta cheese

½ cup marinara sauce

Preparation Method:

Preheat the oven to 375°F (190°C).

Remove stems from mushrooms and place them on a baking sheet.

In a bowl, combine ground turkey, spinach, ricotta cheese, salt, and pepper.

Stuff the mixture into the mushrooms and top with marinara sauce.

Bake for about twenty five minutes until mushrooms turns tender.

Nutritional Information (per serving):

Calories: 310 kcal

Protein: 35 g

Fat: 15 g

Carbohydrates: 10 g

Fibre: 4 g

Baked Cod with Tomato and Olive Salsa

Ingredients (Serves 2):

2 (6 oz) cod fillets

1 cup cherry tomatoes, halved

¼ cup black olives, sliced

2 tbsp olive oil

1 tbsp balsamic vinegar

1 tbsp fresh basil, chopped

Salt and pepper to taste

Preparation Method:

Preheat the oven to 400°F (200°C).

Place cod fillets on a baking sheet and drizzle with olive oil.

In a bowl, mix tomatoes, olives, balsamic vinegar, basil, salt, and pepper.

Spoon the salsa over the cod and bake for 15-20 minutes until cooked through.

Nutritional Information (per serving):

Calories: 330 kcal

Protein: 34 g

Fat: 20 g

Carbohydrates: 5 g

Fibre: 2 g

Creamy Avocado and Chickpea Pasta

Ingredients (Serves 2):

8 oz whole grain pasta

One can (15 oz) of drained and rinsed chickpeas

1 avocado

2 cloves garlic

2 tbsp lemon juice

Salt and pepper to taste

Preparation Method:

Cook pasta according to package instructions; drain.

In a blender, combine avocado, chickpeas, garlic, lemon juice, salt, and pepper; blend until smooth.

Toss the sauce with the pasta and serve.

Nutritional Information (per serving):

Calories: 460 kcal

Protein: 16 g

Fat: 19 g

Carbohydrates: 63 g

Fibre: 10 g

Eggplant and Tomato Stew

Ingredients (Serves 4):

1 large eggplant, diced

2 cups diced tomatoes (canned or fresh)

1 onion, chopped

2 cloves garlic, minced

1 tsp dried oregano

Salt and pepper to taste

Preparation Method:

In a pot, cook onion and garlic until tender.

Add eggplant and cook until slightly softened.

Stir in diced tomatoes, oregano, salt, and pepper. Simmer for 20 minutes.

Nutritional Information (per serving):

Calories: 160 kcal

Protein: 4 g

Fat: 6 g

Carbohydrates: 24 g

Fibre: 9 g

Sesame Crusted Tofu with Broccoli

Ingredients (Serves 2):

1 block (14 oz) firm tofu, pressed and sliced

¼ cup sesame seeds

2 cups broccoli florets

2 tbsp soy sauce

2 tbsp olive oil

Preparation Method:

Preheat oven to 375°F (190°C).

Coat tofu slices with soy sauce and then dip in sesame seeds.

Place on a baking sheet and bake for 25–30 minutes until golden.

Steam broccoli and serve alongside tofu.

Nutritional Information (per serving):

Calories: 320 kcal

Protein: 22 g

Fat: 20 g

Carbohydrates: 18 g

Fibre: 6 g

Roasted Chicken Thighs with Brussels Sprouts

Ingredients (Serves 2):

4 chicken thighs, bone-in, skin-on

2 cups Brussels sprouts, halved

2 tbsp olive oil

1 tsp garlic powder

Salt and pepper to taste

Preparation Method:

Preheat the oven to 400°F (200°C).

In a large bowl, toss chicken thighs and Brussels sprouts with olive oil, garlic powder, salt, and pepper.

Place on a baking sheet and roast for 35-40 minutes until chicken is cooked through and Brussels are crispy.

Nutritional Information (per serving):

Calories: 450 kcal

Protein: 30 g

Fat: 30 g

Carbohydrates: 12 g

Fibre: 5 g

Thai Coconut Curry with Vegetables

Ingredients (Serves 4):

1 can (14 oz) coconut milk

Two cups of mixed vegetables (bell peppers, zucchini, carrots)

2 tbsp red curry paste

1 tbsp fish sauce (or soy sauce for a vegan option)

2 cups cooked brown rice

Preparation Method:

In a pot, heat coconut milk over medium heat and stir in curry paste.

Add mixed vegetables and fish sauce; simmer for 10-15 minutes until veggies are tender.

Serve over cooked brown rice.

Nutritional Information (per serving):

Calories: 400 kcal

Protein: 8 g

Fat: 20 g

Carbohydrates: 52 g

Fibre: 5 g

Chapter 6: Snacks and Desserts for Menopause

Chia Seed Pudding with Berries

Ingredients (Serves 2):

½ cup chia seeds

2 cups almond milk

1 tsp vanilla extract

1 tbsp maple syrup (optional)

1 cup mixed berries (strawberries, blueberries, raspberries)

Preparation Method:

In a bowl, have the chia seeds, almond milk, vanilla extract, and maple syrup combined.

Stir well and refrigerate for at least 4 hours or overnight until thickened.

Serve topped with mixed berries.

Nutritional Information (per serving):

Calories: 280 kcal

Protein: 9 g

Fat: 12 g

Carbohydrates: 36 g

Fibre: 16 g

Almond Flour Muffins

Ingredients (Makes 12 muffins):

2 cups almond flour

½ cup honey or maple syrup

4 eggs

1 tsp baking soda

½ tsp salt

1 tsp cinnamon

Preparation Method:

Preheat the oven to 350°F (175°C) and get a muffin tin lined with liners.

In a bowl, mix almond flour, baking soda, salt, and cinnamon.

In another bowl, whisk together honey, eggs, and dry ingredients.

Get the batter divided into muffin cups and bake for 18-20 minutes.

Nutritional Information (per muffin):

Calories: 130 kcal

Protein: 5 g

Fat: 8 g

Carbohydrates: 12 g

Fibre: 2 g

Greek Yoghourt Parfait

Ingredients (Serves 2):

2 cups Greek yoghourt (unsweetened)

1 cup granola

1 cup sliced fruits (bananas, strawberries, or peaches)

2 tbsp honey (optional)

Preparation Method:

In a glass, layer Greek yoghourt, granola, and sliced fruits.

Drizzle with honey if desired. Serve immediately.

Nutritional Information (per serving):

Calories: 350 kcal

Protein: 20 g

Fat: 8 g

Carbohydrates: 54 g

Fibre: 5 g

Spicy Roasted Chickpeas

Ingredients (Serves 4):

One can (15 oz) of drained rinsed chickpeas

1 tbsp olive oil

1 tsp paprika

½ tsp cumin

Salt and pepper to taste

Preparation Method:

Preheat the oven to 400°F (200°C).

Have the chickpeas tossed with olive oil, paprika, cumin, salt, and pepper.

Spread on a baking sheet and roast for about thirty minutes until it turns crispy.

Nutritional Information (per serving):

Calories: 180 kcal

Protein: 8 g

Fat: 5 g

Carbohydrates: 27 g

Fibre: 8 g

Coconut Macaroons

Ingredients (Makes 12 macaroons):

2 cups shredded unsweetened coconut

½ cup almond flour

½ cup honey or maple syrup

2 egg whites

1 tsp vanilla extract

Preparation Method:

Preheat the oven to 325°F (160°C) and have a baking sheet lined with parchment paper.

In a bowl, mix coconut, almond flour, honey, egg whites, and vanilla.

Drop spoonfuls onto the baking sheet and bake for 15-20 minutes until golden.

Nutritional Information (per macaroon):

Calories: 100 kcal

Protein: 2 g

Fat: 5 g

Carbohydrates: 12 g

Fibre: 2 g

Dark Chocolate-Covered Almonds

Ingredients (Serves 4):

1 cup raw almonds

½ cup dark chocolate chips (70% cocoa or more)

Sea salt (optional)

Preparation Method:

Melt dark chocolate in a microwave or double boiler.

Dip almonds in melted chocolate and place on parchment paper.

Sprinkle with sea salt if desired and let cool until chocolate hardens.

Nutritional Information (per serving):

Calories: 200 kcal

Protein: 6 g

Fat: 17 g

Carbohydrates: 12 g

Fibre: 5 g

Apple Cinnamon Oatmeal Balls

Ingredients (Makes 10 balls):

1 cup rolled oats

½ cup almond butter

½ cup diced apples

1 tsp cinnamon

2 tbsp honey

Preparation Method:

In a bowl, mix all ingredients until well combined.

Roll into small balls and refrigerate for at least 30 minutes before serving.

Nutritional Information (per ball):

Calories: 90 kcal

Protein: 3 g

Fat: 4 g

Carbohydrates: 12 g

Fibre: 2 g

Frozen Yogurt Bark with Fruits

Ingredients (Serves 4):

2 cups Greek yoghourt (plain or flavoured)

1 cup mixed fruits (berries, banana slices, kiwi)

2 tbsp honey (optional)

¼ cup chopped nuts (optional)

Preparation Method:

Spread Greek yoghourt on a baking sheet lined with parchment paper.

Top with mixed fruits, honey, and nuts.

Freeze for at least 4 hours, then break into pieces.

Nutritional Information (per serving):

Calories: 150 kcal

Protein: 10 g

Fat: 4 g

Carbohydrates: 20 g

Fibre: 3 g

Avocado Toast with Seeds

Ingredients (Serves 2):

2 slices whole grain bread

1 ripe avocado

2 tbsp pumpkin seeds

Salt, pepper, and lemon juice to taste

Preparation Method:

Toast the bread slices.

Mash avocado and season with salt, pepper, and lemon juice.

Spread avocado on toast and sprinkle with pumpkin seeds.

Nutritional Information (per serving):

Calories: 250 kcal

Protein: 6 g

Fat: 15 g

Carbohydrates: 27 g

Fibre: 10 g

Peanut Butter Banana Smoothie

Ingredients (Serves 2):

1 ripe banana

2 cups almond milk

2 tbsp peanut butter

1 tbsp honey (optional)

1 tsp ground flaxseed

Preparation Method:

Blend all ingredients until smooth.

Serve immediately, garnished with extra banana slices if desired.

Nutritional Information (per serving):

Calories: 300 kcal

Protein: 10 g

Fat: 12 g

Carbohydrates: 40 g

Fibre: 5 g

Honey and Walnut Stuffed Dates

Ingredients (Serves 4):

12 Medjool dates, pitted

½ cup walnuts, chopped

2 tbsp honey

Preparation Method:

Preheat the oven to 350°F (175°C).

Stuff each date with walnuts and drizzle with honey.

Bake for 10-15 minutes until warm.

Nutritional Information (per serving):

Calories: 190 kcal

Protein: 3 g

Fat: 7 g

Carbohydrates: 31 g

Fibre: 3 g

Cucumber and Hummus Bites

Ingredients (Serves 4):

1 large cucumber, sliced into rounds

1 cup hummus

¼ tsp paprika for garnish

Preparation Method:

Spread hummus on each cucumber slice.

Sprinkle with paprika before serving.

Nutritional Information (per serving):

Calories: 80 kcal

Protein: 3 g

Fat: 4 g

Carbohydrates: 10 g

Fibre: 2 g

Baked Sweet Potato Fries

Ingredients (Serves 4):

2 medium sweet potatoes, cut into fries

2 tbsp olive oil

1 tsp paprika

Salt to taste

Preparation Method:

Preheat the oven to 425°F (220°C).

Get the sweet potato fries tossed with olive oil, paprika, and salt.

Have it spread on a baking sheet and bake for 25-30 minutes until crispy.

Nutritional Information (per serving):

Calories: 150 kcal

Protein: 2 g

Fat: 6 g

Carbohydrates: 22 g

Fibre: 4 g

Matcha Energy Bites

Ingredients (Makes 12 bites):

1 cup oats

¼ cup almond butter

¼ cup honey

1 tbsp matcha powder

¼ cup shredded coconut

Preparation Method:

Mix all ingredients in a bowl until combined.

Roll into bite-sized balls and refrigerate for 30 minutes before serving.

Nutritional Information (per bite):

Calories: 90 kcal

Protein: 3 g

Fat: 4 g

Carbohydrates: 11 g

Fibre: 2 g

Baked Apples with Cinnamon

Ingredients (Serves 4):

4 medium apples, cored

4 tbsp raisins

4 tbsp chopped nuts (walnuts or pecans)

2 tsp cinnamon

2 tbsp honey

Preparation Method:

Preheat the oven to 350°F (175°C).

Stuff each apple with raisins and nuts, then sprinkle with cinnamon.

Drizzle with honey and bake for 25-30 minutes until tender.

Nutritional Information (per serving):

Calories: 160 kcal

Protein: 2 g

Fat: 5 g

Carbohydrates: 28 g

Fibre: 4 g

Chapter 7: Protein-Packed Smoothies and Juices

Banana Almond Protein Smoothie

Ingredients (Serves 2):

2 ripe bananas

2 cups almond milk

4 tbsp almond butter

1 tbsp chia seeds

1 tsp honey (optional)

Preparation Method:

In a blender, combine bananas, almond milk, almond butter, chia seeds, and honey.

Blend until smooth and creamy.

Serve immediately.

Nutritional Information (per serving):

Calories: 320 kcal

Protein: 9 g

Fat: 15 g

Carbohydrates: 45 g

Fibre: 7 g

Berry Spinach Protein Smoothie

Ingredients (Serves 2):

1 cup spinach (fresh)

1 cup mixed berries (frozen or fresh)

1 banana

2 cups Greek yoghourt (plain)

1 tbsp honey (optional)

Preparation Method:

Combine spinach, mixed berries, banana, Greek yoghourt, and honey in a blender.

Blend until smooth and serve.

Nutritional Information (per serving):

Calories: 290 kcal

Protein: 18 g

Fat: 3 g

Carbohydrates: 40 g

Fibre: 5 g

Peanut Butter Banana Smoothie

Ingredients (Serves 2):

2 ripe bananas

2 cups almond milk

4 tbsp peanut butter

1 tbsp flaxseed meal

1 tsp vanilla extract

Preparation Method:

In a blender, combine bananas, almond milk, peanut butter, flaxseed meal, and vanilla.

Blend until smooth and creamy.

Pour into glasses and serve.

Nutritional Information (per serving):

Calories: 350 kcal

Protein: 12 g

Fat: 17 g

Carbohydrates: 40 g

Fibre: 6 g

Tropical Green Protein Smoothie

Ingredients (Serves 2):

1 cup kale (fresh)

1 cup pineapple chunks (fresh or frozen)

1 banana

2 cups coconut water

2 tbsp hemp seeds

Preparation Method:

Add kale, pineapple, banana, coconut water, and hemp seeds to a blender.

Blend until smooth and serve immediately.

Nutritional Information (per serving):

Calories: 230 kcal

Protein: 6 g

Fat: 5 g

Carbohydrates: 47 g

Fibre: 4 g

Chocolate Protein Smoothie

Ingredients (Serves 2):

2 cups almond milk

2 scoops chocolate protein powder

2 tbsp almond butter

1 banana

1 tbsp cacao nibs (for topping)

Preparation Method:

In a blender, combine almond milk, protein powder, almond butter, and banana.

Blend until smooth and pour into glasses.

Top with cacao nibs before serving.

Nutritional Information (per serving):

Calories: 400 kcal

Protein: 28 g

Fat: 15 g

Carbohydrates: 37 g

Fibre: 5 g

Avocado and Spinach Smoothie

Ingredients (Serves 2):

1 ripe avocado

1 cup spinach (fresh)

1 cup almond milk

1 banana

1 tbsp chia seeds

Preparation Method:

In a blender, combine avocado, spinach, almond milk, banana, and chia seeds.

Blend until smooth and creamy.

Serve chilled.

Nutritional Information (per serving):

Calories: 320 kcal

Protein: 7 g

Fat: 18 g

Carbohydrates: 38 g

Fibre: 12 g

Apple Cinnamon Protein Smoothie

Ingredients (Serves 2):

2 apples (cored and chopped)

2 cups almond milk

1 scoop vanilla protein powder

1 tsp cinnamon

1 tbsp almond butter

Preparation Method:

Combine apples, almond milk, protein powder, cinnamon, and almond butter in a blender.

Blend until smooth and serve.

Nutritional Information (per serving):

Calories: 250 kcal

Protein: 12 g

Fat: 8 g

Carbohydrates: 40 g

Fibre: 6 g

Matcha Green Tea Protein Smoothie

Ingredients (Serves 2):

2 cups unsweetened almond milk

2 tsp matcha powder

1 banana

1 scoop vanilla protein powder

2 tbsp chia seeds

Preparation Method:

Blend almond milk, matcha powder, banana, protein powder, and chia seeds until smooth.

Serve immediately.

Nutritional Information (per serving):

Calories: 230 kcal

Protein: 14 g

Fat: 5 g

Carbohydrates: 35 g

Fibre: 8 g

Berry Protein Smoothie Bowl

Ingredients (Serves 2):

1 cup mixed berries (frozen)

1 banana

1 cup Greek yoghourt

1 scoop vanilla protein powder

Toppings: sliced fruits, granola, nuts, and seeds

Preparation Method:

Blend mixed berries, banana, Greek yoghourt, and protein powder until thick and creamy.

Pour into bowls and top with your favourite toppings.

Nutritional Information (per serving):

Calories: 300 kcal

Protein: 20 g

Fat: 5 g

Carbohydrates: 50 g

Fibre: 6 g

Cocoa Almond Protein Smoothie

Ingredients (Serves 2):

2 cups almond milk

2 tbsp cocoa powder

2 scoops vanilla protein powder

1 banana

1 tbsp almond butter

Preparation Method:

Combine almond milk, cocoa powder, protein powder, banana, and almond butter in a blender.

Blend until smooth and serve.

Nutritional Information (per serving):

Calories: 350 kcal

Protein: 25 g

Fat: 12 g

Carbohydrates: 35 g

Fibre: 6 g

Cucumber Mint Green Juice

Ingredients (Serves 2):

1 large cucumber

1 cup spinach (fresh)

1 green apple

1 lemon (juiced)

A handful of fresh mint leaves

Preparation Method:

Juice the cucumber, spinach, apple, and mint leaves using a juicer.

Stir in fresh lemon juice and serve chilled.

Nutritional Information (per serving):

Calories: 70 kcal

Protein: 2 g

Fat: 0 g

Carbohydrates: 16 g

Fibre: 2 g

Tropical Protein Juice

Ingredients (Serves 2):

1 cup pineapple chunks

1 orange (peeled)

1 cup coconut water

1 scoop vanilla protein powder

Preparation Method:

Blend pineapple, orange, coconut water, and protein powder until smooth. Serve chilled.

Nutritional Information (per serving):

Calories: 210 kcal

Protein: 10 g

Fat: 0 g

Carbohydrates: 45 g

Fibre: 5 g

Strawberry Banana Protein Smoothie

Ingredients (Serves 2):

1 cup strawberries (fresh or frozen)

1 banana

2 cups almond milk

2 scoops vanilla protein powder

1 tbsp chia seeds

Preparation Method:

Blend strawberries, banana, almond milk, protein powder, and chia seeds until smooth.

Serve immediately.

Nutritional Information (per serving):

Calories: 290 kcal

Protein: 20 g

Fat: 4 g

Carbohydrates: 45 g

Fibre: 7 g

Chocolate Peanut Butter Protein Shake

Ingredients (Serves 2):

2 cups almond milk

2 scoops chocolate protein powder

4 tbsp peanut butter

1 banana

Ice cubes (optional)

Preparation Method:

Combine almond milk, protein powder, peanut butter, and banana in a blender.

Blend until smooth and serve over ice if desired.

Nutritional Information (per serving):

Calories: 410 kcal

Protein: 28 g

Fat: 18 g

Carbohydrates: 36 g

Fibre: 5 g

Berry Coconut Protein Smoothie

Ingredients (Serves 2):

1 cup mixed berries (frozen or fresh)

1 cup coconut milk

1 scoop vanilla protein powder

1 tbsp shredded coconut

1 tsp honey (optional)

Preparation Method:

Blend mixed berries, coconut milk, protein powder, shredded coconut, and honey until smooth.

Serve immediately.

Nutritional Information (per serving):

Calories: 260 kcal

Protein: 15 g

Fat: 12 g

Carbohydrates: 28 g

Fibre: 5 g

Chapter 8 – Bonus: 30-Day Next Level Meal Plan

Day 1 to 7

Day 1

Breakfast: Spinach and Feta Omelet

Lunch: Grilled Chicken Salad with Avocado and Lime Dressing

Dinner: Salmon with Quinoa and Steamed Broccoli

Snack: Almond Butter and Celery Sticks

Smoothie: Berry Coconut Protein Smoothie

Day 2

Breakfast: Greek Yogurt Parfait with Berries and Nuts

Lunch: Turkey Lettuce Wraps with Avocado

Dinner: Stir-Fried Tofu with Vegetables

Snack: Hummus with Baby Carrots

Smoothie: Spinach and Banana Protein Smoothie

Day 3

Breakfast: Chia Seed Pudding with Almond Milk and Berries

Lunch: Quinoa Salad with Chickpeas and Veggies

Dinner: Grilled Shrimp with Zucchini Noodles

Snack: Sliced Apple with Peanut Butter

Smoothie: Mango Coconut Protein Smoothie

Day 4

Breakfast: Avocado Toast with Poached Egg

Lunch: Beef and Broccoli Stir-Fry

Dinner: Baked Cod with Sweet Potato Mash

Snack: Greek Yoghourt with Honey

Smoothie: Strawberry Banana Protein Smoothie

Day 5

Breakfast: Oatmeal with Chia Seeds and Almonds

Lunch: Spinach and Turkey Wrap

Dinner: Chicken Thighs with Roasted Brussels Sprouts

Snack: Dark Chocolate Almonds

Smoothie: Green Apple and Kale Protein Smoothie

Day 6

Breakfast: Scrambled Eggs with Salsa and Avocado

Lunch: Tuna Salad with Mixed Greens

Dinner: Grilled Eggplant with Tomato Sauce and Mozzarella

Snack: Rice Cakes with Almond Butter

Smoothie: Chocolate Peanut Butter Protein Smoothie

Day 7

Breakfast: Smoothie Bowl with Berries and Granola

Lunch: Quinoa and Black Bean Bowl

Dinner: Lemon Herb Chicken with Asparagus

Snack: Cottage Cheese with Pineapple

Smoothie: Tropical Green Protein Smoothie

Day 8 to 14

Day 8

Breakfast: Whole Grain Pancakes with Berries

Lunch: Lentil Soup with Whole Grain Bread

Dinner: Grilled Salmon with Spinach Salad

Snack: Mixed Nuts

Smoothie: Berry Spinach Protein Smoothie

Day 9

Breakfast: Egg and Veggie Muffins

Lunch: Chicken Caesar Salad (low-carb)

Dinner: Beef Tacos with Lettuce Wraps

Snack: Cucumber Slices with Hummus

Smoothie: Berry Coconut Protein Smoothie

Day 10

Breakfast: Almond Flour Muffins

Lunch: Shrimp and Avocado Salad

Dinner: Stuffed Bell Peppers with Ground Turkey

Snack: Hard-Boiled Eggs

Smoothie: Chocolate Banana Protein Smoothie

Day 11

Breakfast: Quinoa Porridge with Almond Milk

Lunch: Spinach Salad with Grilled Chicken

Dinner: Baked Lemon Herb Cod with Veggies

Snack: Dark Chocolate Covered Strawberries

Smoothie: Vanilla Berry Protein Smoothie

Day 12

Breakfast: Savory Oatmeal with Eggs and Avocado

Lunch: Turkey and Avocado Salad

Dinner: Grilled Lamb Chops with Green Beans

Snack: Cheese and Crackers

Smoothie: Kale and Apple Protein Smoothie

Day 13

Breakfast: Protein Pancakes with Berries

Lunch: Greek Salad with Grilled Chicken

Dinner: Zucchini Lasagna

Snack: Sliced Bell Peppers with Guacamole

Smoothie: Chocolate Mint Protein Smoothie

Day 14

Breakfast: Smoothie Bowl with Granola and Fruit

Lunch: Baked Chicken with Sweet Potato

Dinner: Grilled Mahi-Mahi with Mango Salsa

Snack: Yogurt with Granola

Smoothie: Orange Carrot Protein Smoothie

Day 15 to 21

Day 15

Breakfast: Overnight Oats with Chia Seeds

Lunch: Falafel Wrap with Hummus

Dinner: Stir-Fried Beef with Broccoli

Snack: Pumpkin Seeds

Smoothie: Berry Green Protein Smoothie

Day 16

Breakfast: Cottage Cheese with Berries and Nuts

Lunch: Chicken and Vegetable Stir-Fry

Dinner: Baked Salmon with Quinoa

Snack: Carrot Sticks with Hummus

Smoothie: Peanut Butter Banana Protein Smoothie

Day 17

Breakfast: Scrambled Eggs with Spinach and Feta

Lunch: Tuna Salad with Mixed Greens

Dinner: Lemon Garlic Shrimp with Zucchini Noodles

Snack: Greek Yoghourt with Honey

Smoothie: Mixed Berry Protein Smoothie

Day 18

Breakfast: Green Smoothie with Spinach and Avocado

Lunch: Chicken Lettuce Wraps

Dinner: Grilled Vegetable Platter with Quinoa

Snack: Almonds and Dark Chocolate

Smoothie: Strawberry Kiwi Protein Smoothie

Day 19

Breakfast: Chia Seed Pudding with Almond Milk

Lunch: Turkey and Veggie Bowl

Dinner: Herb-Roasted Chicken with Sweet Potatoes

Snack: Sliced Apple with Almond Butter

Smoothie: Chocolate Cherry Protein Smoothie

Day 20

Breakfast: Protein Smoothie Bowl

Lunch: Shrimp and Quinoa Salad

Dinner: Grilled Pork Chops with Roasted Vegetables

Snack: Cheese Sticks

Smoothie: Vanilla Berry Protein Smoothie

Day 21

Breakfast: Smoothie with Spinach and Protein Powder

Lunch: Mediterranean Quinoa Salad

Dinner: Lemon Thyme Baked Chicken

Snack: Hummus with Carrot Sticks

Smoothie: Tropical Green Protein Smoothie

Day 22 to 30

Day 22

Breakfast: Oatmeal with Almonds and Berries

Lunch: Chicken Salad with Nuts

Dinner: Baked Halibut with Asparagus

Snack: Yogurt with Seeds

Smoothie: Berry Mango Protein Smoothie

Day 23

Breakfast: Protein-Packed Smoothie

Lunch: Lentil Salad with Vegetables

Dinner: Grilled Chicken with Cauliflower Rice

Snack: Nut Mix

Smoothie: Chocolate Peanut Butter Protein Smoothie

Day 24

Breakfast: Egg Muffins with Spinach

Lunch: Beef and Veggie Stir-Fry

Dinner: Zucchini Noodles with Marinara and Meatballs

Snack: Apple with Almond Butter

Smoothie: Berry Avocado Protein Smoothie

Day 25

Breakfast: Chia Seed and Almond Milk Pudding

Lunch: Tuna Salad on Greens

Dinner: Herb-Roasted Chicken with Brussels Sprouts

Snack: Cucumber with Hummus

Smoothie: Vanilla Berry Protein Smoothie

Day 26
Breakfast: Smoothie Bowl with Granola
Lunch: Grilled Vegetable Salad
Dinner: Lemon Garlic Shrimp with Veggies
Snack: Dark Chocolate Almonds
Smoothie: Mixed Berry Protein Smoothie

Day 27
Breakfast: Scrambled Eggs with Tomatoes and Spinach
Lunch: Grilled Chicken Caesar Salad
Dinner: Beef Tacos with Lettuce Wraps
Snack: Greek Yoghourt with Nuts
Smoothie: Strawberry Banana Protein Smoothie

Day 28
Breakfast: Oatmeal with Walnuts and Berries
Lunch: Quinoa Bowl with Chickpeas
Dinner: Baked Salmon with Vegetables
Snack: Hard-Boiled Eggs
Smoothie: Tropical Green Protein Smoothie

Day 29
Breakfast: Cottage Cheese with Fruits
Lunch: Turkey and Avocado Salad
Dinner: Grilled Shrimp with Zucchini Noodles
Snack: Sliced Veggies with Dip
Smoothie: Chocolate Mint Protein Smoothie

Day 30
Breakfast: Smoothie with Spinach and Protein Powder
Lunch: Mediterranean Chickpea Salad
Dinner: Herb-Roasted Chicken with Sweet Potato
Snack: Mixed Nuts
Smoothie: Berry Protein Smoothie

Conclusion

Redefining Your Strength: Thriving in Menopause and Beyond

As you reach this chapter of life known as menopause, it is essential to embrace the changes and transformations that come with it. This transition can feel daunting; however, it also represents an incredible opportunity for growth, self-discovery, and empowerment. The narrative around menopause is shifting from one of loss and decline to a powerful affirmation of strength and vitality. This is your time to redefine what strength means for you, both physically and emotionally, as you step into the next level of your life.

Menopause is often portrayed negatively in popular culture—characterised by weight gain, mood swings, and the fear of ageing. Yet, within this biological transition lies a chance to cultivate resilience and foster a deeper understanding of your body and its needs. With the right mindset and tools, you can thrive during this stage of life, ensuring that it becomes a period of renewal rather than resignation.

The foundation for thriving in menopause starts with knowledge. Understanding the hormonal changes taking place in your body is crucial. These hormonal shifts, while they can lead to various symptoms, are also your body's way of signalling that it's time to make adjustments—both in lifestyle and self-care practices. This cookbook serves as a guide, offering you recipes and nutritional insights designed to support your journey through menopause and beyond. The focus on high-protein, low-carb meals, rich in omega-3 fatty acids and antioxidants, will help mitigate the symptoms of menopause while enhancing your overall health and well-being.

It is essential to recognize that your nutritional needs evolve during menopause. Your metabolism may slow, requiring you to reassess your dietary choices to maintain optimal health and energy levels. This is where the culinary creativity in this book can empower you. The recipes provided are not just about sustenance; they are about nourishing your body with purpose and intention. Each meal has been thoughtfully designed to support hormone balance, provide sustained energy, and fortify your physical strength. Incorporating nutrient-dense foods such as leafy greens, lean proteins, healthy fats, and fibre-rich whole grains will help you navigate this transition with grace and vitality.

Moreover, physical activity plays a vital role in managing menopausal symptoms and enhancing overall health. The workouts and fitness recommendations you explore in this book can help you adapt your exercise routine to better align with your changing body. Engaging in strength training, flexibility exercises, and cardiovascular workouts will not only improve your physical strength but also elevate your mood and boost your confidence. Exercise is not just a tool for weight management; it is a pathway to resilience, vitality, and joy during this transformative stage of life.

It's also crucial to prioritise self-care and mental wellness as you journey through menopause. Acknowledging your emotional and psychological needs is just as important as tending to your physical health. Embrace practices such as mindfulness, meditation, or yoga to foster a positive mindset. Surround yourself with supportive friends and loved ones who understand and respect your journey. Sharing your experiences can lead to connections that empower you to face the challenges of menopause with courage and positivity.

As you redefine your strength during menopause, remember that you are not alone. Many women are walking this path and thriving in their unique ways. By fostering a community of support and sharing experiences, you can inspire one another to embrace this new phase of life with enthusiasm and determination.

Final Words of Encouragement for the Next Level

In closing, I want to leave you with a message of encouragement: Menopause is not an end but a beginning. It is an invitation to explore the depths of your strength and resilience, to nurture your body and mind with intention, and to celebrate the wisdom that comes with age. Each chapter of your life has prepared you for this moment; you are equipped with the tools, knowledge, and experiences to navigate it successfully.

This cookbook is not just a collection of recipes; it is a manifesto for embracing your health and well-being during menopause. It is a reminder that nourishing your body can lead to transformative experiences, both inside and out.

As you embark on this journey, I encourage you to experiment with the recipes, savour the flavours, and pay attention to how the foods you consume affect your energy levels, mood, and overall health. Use this opportunity to discover new ingredients, explore culinary techniques, and foster a joyful relationship with food that honours your body and its needs.

Remember, thriving in menopause is possible. By adopting a proactive approach to your health, fostering a supportive community, and maintaining an open mind, you can navigate this chapter with grace and confidence. Redefine your narrative, embrace the changes, and step into this new phase of life with a sense of purpose and empowerment.

The next level of your life awaits—filled with promise, potential, and newfound strength. Embrace it wholeheartedly, knowing that you have the power to thrive during menopause and beyond.

4 BOOKS BONUS GIFTS

Please scan each QR code one by one, and you'll be directed to a website where you can claim your free books. Whenever you're prompted to enter a price, simply input "$0," as these books are completely free for you.

BONUS 2
50 JUICES

BONUS 3
50 SMOOTHIES

BONUS 4
50 SNACKS

BONUS 5
50 DESSERTS

Printed in Great Britain
by Amazon

51195639R00068